Vegan Diet

Combining and Understanding a Vegetarian and Keto Diet Lifestyle

(Plant based diet recipes including delicious vegan meals)

Jose Smith

Published by Robert Satterfield
Publishing House

© **Jose Smith**

All Rights Reserved

Vegan Diet Recipes Cookbook: Combining and Understanding a Vegetarian and Keto Diet Lifestyle (Plant based diet recipes including delicious vegan meals)

ISBN 978-1-989682-94-4

Legal & Disclaimer

The information contained in this book is not designed to replace or take the place of any form of medicine or professional medical advice. The information in this book has been provided for educational and entertainment purposes only.

TABLE OF CONTENT

Part 1

Introduction

This vegan breakfast cookbook contains a huge variety of vegan breakfast recipes that are 100% vegan!

If you are a vegan struggling to find some decent great tasting breakfast recipes, then you will love this cookbook. These recipes were hand picked from my collection, and were selected not only because they are vegan but because they are easy recipes that anyone can make. Like most vegan recipes, these breakfast recipes are also very healthy and nutritious.

We hope you enjoy this vegan breakfast cookbook!

Apple Carrot Breakfast Muffins

Ingredients
1 cup brown sugar
1/2 cup white sugar
2 1/2 cups all-purpose flour
4 teaspoons baking soda
1 teaspoon baking powder
4 teaspoons ground cinnamon
2 teaspoons salt
2 cups finely grated carrots
2 large apples - peeled, cored and shredded
6 teaspoons egg replacer (dry)
1 1/4 cups applesauce
1/4 cup vegetable oil

Directions
Preheat oven to 375 degrees F (190 degrees C). Grease muffin cups or line with paper muffin liners.

In a large bowl combine brown sugar, white sugar, flour, baking soda, baking powder, cinnamon and salt. Stir in carrot and apple; mix well.

In a small bowl whisk together egg substitute, applesauce and oil. Stir into dry ingredients.

Spoon batter into prepared pans.

Bake in preheated oven for 20 minutes. Let muffins cool in pan for 5 minutes before removing from pans to cool completely.

Pumpkin Pancakes

Ingredients
2 1/2 cups whole wheat flour
2 1/2 cups water
1/2 cup soy milk
2 tbsp baking powder
1 tsp salt
1/2 cup mashed, cooked pumpkin
1/2 tsp cinnamon
1/4 tsp nutmeg
1/4 tsp allspice

1 tsp vanilla extract
1/2 tsp baking soda
1 tsp apple cider vinegar

Directions

Combine soymilk with the tsp vinegar in a separate bowl. Allow 5 minutes for it to curdle.

Stir together pumpkin, spices, water and soymilk in mixing bowl.

Add in remaining Ingredients and stir until just moist, and stop stirring.

Let sit 5 minutes to rise and lightly stir again. Let rest 5 more minutes. Pour in a frying pan or skillet.

Cook pancakes on stove and serve.

Maple Oatmeal

Ingredients
3/4 cup water
1/4 cup steel-cut oats
1 tablespoon natural peanut butter
1 tablespoon maple syrup
1/2 teaspoon brown sugar

Directions
Bring water to a boil in a saucepan, stir steel cut oats into water, and reduce heat to medium-low.

Cover and cook until oats are tender, 5 to 7 minutes, stirring occasionally. Remove from heat and let stand 1 minute.

Stir peanut butter, maple syrup, and brown sugar into oats.

Apple Pancakes

Ingredients
2 cups whole wheat flour
2 apples, peeled and cored
1 1/2 cups almond milk
1/2 cup coconut oil, melted
1/4 cup water
2 tablespoons baking powder
2 tablespoons cane sugar, or to taste
1 teaspoon ground nutmeg
1/2 teaspoon ground cinnamon

Directions
Blend flour, apples, almond milk, coconut oil, water, baking powder, cane sugar, nutmeg, and cinnamon in a blender until smooth.

Heat a non-stick griddle over medium-high heat. Drop batter by large spoonfuls onto the griddle and cook until bubbles form and the edges are dry, 3 to 4 minutes.

Flip and cook until browned on the other side, 2 to 3 minutes. Repeat with remaining batter.

Vegan French Toast

Ingredients
1 cup soy milk
2 tablespoons all-purpose flour
1 tablespoon nutritional yeast
1 teaspoon raw sugar
1 teaspoon vanilla extract
1/3 teaspoon ground cinnamon
4 slices vegan bread

Directions
Whisk soy milk, flour, nutritional yeast, sugar, vanilla extract, and cinnamon together in a bowl; transfer to a rimmed plate or shallow dish. Dip both sides of each bread slice in soy milk mixture.

Heat a lightly oiled skillet over medium-low heat.

Cook each slice of bread until golden brown, 3 to 4 minutes per side.

Easy Vegan Breakfast Skillet

Ingredients
2 cups frozen hash browns
1 cup chopped onion
1 cup chopped bell pepper
1 cup chopped broccoli
1 12-oz. package firm tofu, crumbled
2 tbsp nutritional yeast
1/2 14-oz package vegan sausages, divided into 4 patties

Directions

Heat a large non-stick skillet to medium-high.

Spray 1/2 of the skillet generously with cooking spray and add the hash browns.

Divide the sausage into patties and add.

Once the potatoes begin to brown, add the onion and continue cooking 5-7 minutes. Flip the sausage patties.

Add bell pepper and broccoli, stir to ensure even cooking.

Save room on the opposite end of the skillet for the tofu. While the vegetables cook, crumble the tofu.

Spray the opposite end of the skillet with cooking spray, and add the tofu.

Sprinkle the tofu with the nutritional yeast.

Scramble the tofu and yeast together to cook off any excess liquid.

Place 1/4 of the potato vegetable mixture on each plate then top with the tofu.

Season as desired.

Breakfast Oatmeal Squares

Ingredients
3cups oatmeal
1cup unsweetened plain almond milk
1/2 cup agave
1/2 cup applesauce
2 mashed ripe bananas
2 tsp baking powder
1 tsp salt
1 tsp vanilla
1 tsp cinnamon

Directions
Mix all Ingredients in a bowl. Pour in greased baking pan. Bake at 350 for 25 minutes.

Easy Vegan Pancakes

Ingredients
4 cups self-rising flour
1 tablespoon white sugar
1 tablespoon custard powder
2 cups soy milk

Directions
In a large bowl, stir together the flour, sugar and custard powder. Mix in the soy milk with a whisk so there are no lumps.

Heat a griddle over medium heat, and coat with nonstick cooking spray. Spoon batter onto the surface, and cook until bubbles begin to form on the surface.

Flip with a spatula and cook on the other side until golden.

Spicy Vegan Breakfast Hash

Ingredients
1 cup frozen hash browns
1/4 onion thinly sliced
1 cup mushrooms
3 cups spinach
1 small or 1/2 medium hot pepper
1 1/2 tbsp nutritional yeast
salt and pepper to taste

Directions
In a small non-stick pan, brown the hash browns.

In a separate pan, saute the onions in oil spray until translucent. Add sliced pepper and sliced mushrooms and saute until mushrooms are tender.

Sprinkle with nutritional yeast, add spinach and a little water, cover and simmer until spinach is cooked. Stir well to incorporate the nutritional yeast

Add salt and pepper to taste.

Banana Blueberry Muffins

Ingredients
2 very ripe bananas, mashed
1/2 cup white sugar
1/2 teaspoon baking powder
1/2 teaspoon salt
3/4 cup all-purpose flour
1/2 cup whole wheat pastry flour
1 1/2 teaspoons egg replacer (dry)
2 tablespoons water
1/2 cup blueberries

Directions
Preheat oven to 350 degrees F (175 degrees C). Grease muffin cups or line with paper muffin liners.

In a large bowl combine mashed bananas, sugar, baking powder, salt and flours; mix until smooth. In a small bowl or cup combine egg replacer and water; stir into banana mixture. Fold in blueberries.

Spoon batter evenly, about 1/4 cup each, into muffin cups.

Bake in preheated oven for 20 to 25 minutes, or until golden brown.

Blueberry Pancakes

Ingredients
1 cup soy milk
1/2 cup water
1 cup whole wheat flour
1/2 cup stone ground cornmeal
1 teaspoon baking powder
1/2 teaspoon baking soda
1/4 teaspoon salt
1 cup fresh blueberries
2 tablespoons vegetable oil

Directions
Preheat oven to 200F.

In a small bowl combine the soy milk and water.

In a large bowl, combine the flour, cornmeal, baking powder, baking soda and salt. Stir in the soy milk mixture just until combined. Fold in the blueberries and let the batter sit for 5 minutes.

Lightly oil a skillet or griddle and heat over medium heat. Pour about 1/4 cup of batter onto the hot griddle and cook until pancakes are bubbly on top and edges are slightly dry looking. Turn and cook until pancakes are browned. Transfer to a baking sheet and keep warm in the oven while cooking the remaining batter.

Vegan Cornbread Muffins

Ingredients
1/2 cup cornmeal
1/2 cup whole-wheat pastry flour

1/2 teaspoon baking soda
1/2 teaspoon salt
1/2 cup applesauce
1/2 cup soy milk
1/4 cup agave nectar
2 tablespoons canola oil

Directions
Preheat oven to 325 degrees F (165 degrees C). Lightly grease a muffin pan.

Combine the cornmeal, flour, baking soda, and salt in a large bowl; stir in the applesauce, soy milk, and agave nectar. Slowly add the oil while stirring. Pour the mixture into the muffin pan.

Bake in the preheated oven until a toothpick or small knife inserted in the crown of a muffin comes out clean, 15 to 20 minutes.

Pumpkin Loaf

Ingredients
2 tablespoons flax seed meal
6 tablespoons water
1 1/2 cups sugar
1 cup canned pumpkin puree
1/2 cup applesauce
1 1/3 cups all-purpose flour
1/3 cup whole wheat pastry flour
1 teaspoon baking soda
1 teaspoon ground cinnamon
3/4 teaspoon salt
1/2 teaspoon baking powder
1/2 teaspoon ground nutmeg
1/4 teaspoon ground cloves

Directions
Preheat oven to 350 degrees F (175 degrees C). Lightly grease one 9x5 inch loaf pan.

Whisk together flax seed meal and water. Mix in sugar, pumpkin and apple sauce.

In a large bowl, stir together all-purpose flour, whole wheat flour, baking soda, cinnamon, salt, baking powder, nutmeg, and cloves. Add flour mixture to pumpkin mixture; stir until smooth. Pour batter into prepared pan.

Bake in preheated oven for 65 to 70 minutes, until a toothpick inserted into center of the loaf comes out clean.

Vegan Waffles

Ingredients
1 cup whole wheat flour
1 cup unbleached white flour
1/2 tsp cinnamon
1 1/2 tsp baking powder
2 tbs granulated sugar
2 cups almond or soy milk
1/3 cup unsweetened apple sauce

Directions
Mix all dry Ingredients in one bowl. Stir together almond milk and apple sauce in a

separate bowl and pour into dry ingredient, stirring gently until blended.

Consistency should be a pourable batter; if too thick, add some more milk.

Cook using a waffle iron.

Vegan Potato Pancakes

Ingredients
10 russet potatoes, peeled and shredded
1 carrot, peeled and shredded
1 onion, finely diced
5 cloves garlic, crushed
1 tablespoon chopped flat leaf parsley
1 tablespoon chopped fresh dill
2 tablespoons fresh lemon juice
1/4 cup olive oil
2 tablespoons all-purpose flour
2 cups dry vegan bread crumbs
salt and pepper to taste
olive oil for frying, as needed

Directions

Mix potatoes, carrot, onion, garlic, parsley, and dill in a large bowl. Stir in lemon juice, 1/4 cup of olive oil, flour, bread crumbs, salt, and pepper. Knead just until mixture holds together.

Heat the remaining 1/4 cup olive oil in a skillet over medium heat. Working in batches, drop spoonfuls of potato mixture in hot oil.

Cook approximately 4 minutes per side, or until golden brown. Serve hot.

Vegan Crepes

Ingredients
1/2 cup soy milk
1/4 cup melted soy margarine

1/2 cup water
1 tablespoon turbinado sugar
2 tablespoons maple syrup
1 cup unbleached all-purpose flour
1/4 teaspoon salt

Directions
In a large mixing bowl, blend soy milk, water, 1/4 cup margarine, sugar, syrup, flour, and salt. Cover and chill the mixture for 2 hours.

Lightly grease a 5 to 6 inch skillet with some soy margarine. Heat the skillet until hot.

Pour approximately 3 tablespoons batter into the skillet. Swirl to make the batter cover the skillet's bottom.

Cook until golden, flip and cook on opposite side.

Banana Oatmeal Porridge

Ingredients
1 3/4 cups water
1/4 teaspoon Himalayan pink salt
1 cup rolled oats
3 large ripe bananas, mashed
3 tablespoons sunflower seed butter
2 tablespoons agave nectar

Directions
Bring water and salt to a boil in a saucepan; add oats and simmer until desired consistency is reached, about 5 minutes.

Remove saucepan from heat and stir in bananas, sunflower seed butter, and agave nectar.

Breakfast Couscous

Ingredients
3/4 cup vanilla soymilk

1/4 cup orange juice
1/2 cup dry couscous
1/2 banana, mashed or sliced
1 tsp cinnamon

Directions
In a small pot on high heat bring the milk and juice to a boil.

Reduce heat and stir in couscous, banana and cinnamon. Cover with lid and simmer for 2-3 minutes.

Turn off heat and let sit for an additional 2 minutes.

Serve immediately. Makes two servings.

Zucchini Banana Muffins

Ingredients
2 1/3 cups grated zucchini

1 1/2 over-ripe bananas, mashed
1 cup applesauce
1 cup brown sugar
1/4 cup vegetable oil
1 tablespoon lemon juice
1 1/2 teaspoons vanilla extract
3 cups all-purpose flour
1 tablespoon baking soda
1 tablespoon ground cinnamon
2 teaspoons ground nutmeg
1 teaspoon baking powder
1 teaspoon salt
1/4 teaspoon ground cloves
1 tablespoon white sugar
1 teaspoon ground cinnamon

Directions
Preheat oven to 350 degrees F (175 degrees C). Grease or line 24 muffin cups with paper liners.
Combine zucchini, bananas, applesauce, brown sugar, oil, lemon juice, and vanilla extract together in a large bowl. Whisk flour, baking soda, 1 tablespoon cinnamon, nutmeg, baking powder, salt, and cloves together in a separate bowl.

Slowly add flour mixture to zucchini mixture while continuously stirring until batter is just combined. Spoon batter into prepared muffin cups about 3/4-full.

Mix white sugar and 1 teaspoon cinnamon together in a small bowl; sprinkle over batter.

Bake in the preheated oven until a toothpick inserted in the center of a muffin comes out clean, about 30 minutes.

Apple Muffins

Ingredients
1 1/4 cups bran flakes cereal
1 1/4 cups all-purpose flour
1/3 cup brown sugar
1 teaspoon ground cinnamon
1 tablespoon baking powder
1 1/4 cups apple juice

1/4 cup margarine, melted
1 teaspoon vanilla extract
1 apple - peeled, cored and chopped

Directions
Preheat oven to 375 F. Grease muffin tins.

In a mixing bowl, combine bran flakes, flour, brown sugar, cinnamon and baking powder. Stir in apple juice, margarine, vanilla, and apple. Spoon the mixture into the greased muffin tins.

Bake at 375 F for 25 to 30 minutes.

Zucchini Chocolate Pancakes

Ingredients
2 tablespoons water
1 tablespoon flax seeds
1/2 cup unsweetened almond milk

1 very ripe banana, mashed
1/4 cup shredded zucchini
1/4 teaspoon vanilla extract
1/2 cup all-purpose flour
1 tablespoon unsweetened cocoa powder
1 1/2 teaspoons Truvia brown sugar baking blend
1/2 teaspoon baking powder
1/4 teaspoon baking soda
1/4 teaspoon ground cinnamon
1 pinch sea salt
cooking spray

Directions
Combine water and flax seeds in a small bowl. Refrigerate until mixture thickens and has an egg-like consistency, 15 to 30 minutes. Stir in almond milk, banana, zucchini, and vanilla extract.

Mix flour, cocoa powder, brown sugar baking blend, baking powder, baking soda, cinnamon, and sea salt together in a bowl. Pour in flax mixture; stir until batter is just combined.

Heat a large griddle over medium heat and spray with cooking spray. Drop 1/3 cup batter onto the griddle and cook until bubbles form and bottoms are golden brown, about 5 minutes.

Flip and cook until browned on the other side, 4 to 6 minutes. Transfer to a baking rack to cool. Repeat with remaining batter.

Coconut Apricot Oatmeal

Ingredients
1 cup water
½ cup old-fashioned rolled oats
½ teaspoon ground cinnamon
6 dried apricots, chopped
1 tablespoon unsweetened shredded coconut

Directions
Combine water, oats and cinnamon in a small saucepan. Bring to a boil over high

heat. Reduce heat to a simmer and cook, stirring occasionally, until creamy, about 5 minutes.

Serve topped with apricots and coconut.

Granola Breakfast

Ingredients
cooking spray
3 cups rolled oats
2/3 cup wheat germ
1/2 cup slivered almonds
1 pinch ground nutmeg
1 1/2 teaspoons ground cinnamon
1/2 cup apple juice
1/2 cup molasses
1 teaspoon vanilla extract
1 cup dried mixed fruit
1 cup quartered dried apricots

Directions

Preheat oven to 350F. Prepare two cookie sheets with cooking spray.

In a large bowl, combine oats, wheat germ, almonds, cinnamon and nutmeg. In a separate bowl, mix apple juice, molasses and extract. Pour the wet Ingredients into the dry ingredients, stirring to coat. Spread mixture onto baking sheets.

Bake for 30 minutes in preheated oven, stirring mixture every 10 to 15 minutes, or until granola has a golden brown color. Let cool. Stir in dried fruit. Store in an airtight container.

Zucchini Walnut Muffins

Ingredients
1/4 cup chia seeds
1 cup water
1 cup cashew flour
1/4 cup ground flax seed

2 tablespoons coconut flour
2 tablespoons tapioca starch
1 tablespoon ground cinnamon
1 teaspoon baking soda
1/2 teaspoon salt
1 cup chopped dates
1 cup chopped walnuts
1 cup shredded zucchini
1/3 cup applesauce
2 tablespoons coconut oil, melted
1 fluid ounce liquid stevia, or to taste

Directions
Preheat oven to 375 F. Line 12 muffin cups with paper liners.

Soak chia seeds in the water in a bowl until thickened and paste-like, 5 to 10 minutes.

Whisk cashew flour, flax seed, coconut flour, tapioca starch, cinnamon, baking soda, and salt together in a bowl.

Mix chia seed mixture, dates, walnuts, zucchini, applesauce, coconut oil, and stevia together in a separate bowl; stir into dry mixture until batter is just combined. Spoon batter into the muffin cups.

Bake in the preheated oven until a toothpick inserted in the middle of a muffin comes out clean, 30 to 35 minutes. Cool muffins in the muffin tin on a wire rack before removing, about 10 minutes; cool another 5 minutes before serving.

Cinnamon Raisin Breakfast Cookies

Ingredients
1 1/3 cup cups oats
4 tablespoons raisins
4 tablespoons flour
1 1/3 cups powdered soy milk
1 cup unsweetened applesauce (no-sugar-added)
1 teaspoon cinnamon
1 teaspoon baking powder
4 tablespoon no-calorie artificial sweetener

Directions

Preheat oven to 350 degrees. Spray a large cookie sheet with cooking spray.

Mix all Ingredients together and spoon on sheet. Bake for 15-20 minutes.

Tofu Breakfast Casserole

Ingredients

1 block extra firm tofu (drained and pressed)
1 small onion chopped
1/2 cup red sweet pepper chopped
2-3 large mushrooms sliced
1 garlic clove minced
2 tbsp nutritional yeast
1.5 tsp ground tumeric
1/2 cup non dairy vegan shredded cheese
1 cup hash browns
1 dash salt
1 tsp black pepper

1.5 tbsp extra virgin olive oil

Directions
Preheat oven to 350F.

In a large mixing bowl crumble tofu with to the look of scrambled eggs. Add garlic powder, tumeric, nutritional yeast - stir to coat and set aside.

In a pan add the olive oil and cook the onions, garlic, mushrooms and peppers until tender but not too soft. Sprinkle with black pepper and dash of salt. Remove from pan and add to the tofu crumbles.

Stir in vegan cheese shreds.

In a casserole dish lay the hashbrowns evenly. Top with the tofu scramble mixture.

Bake at 350F for approx. 30 minutes. Remove from oven and serve.

Banana Muffins

Ingredients
3 cups all-purpose flour
1 cup white sugar
1/2 cup brown sugar
2 teaspoons ground cinnamon
2 teaspoons baking powder
1 teaspoon baking soda
1 teaspoon ground nutmeg
1 teaspoon salt
2 cups mashed ripe bananas
1 cup canola oil
1 cup coconut milk

Directions
Preheat oven to 350 degrees F (175 degrees C). Grease 12 muffin cups or line with paper liners.

Mix flour, white sugar, brown sugar, cinnamon, baking powder, baking soda, nutmeg, and salt together in a large bowl.

Stir bananas, canola oil, and coconut milk together in a separate bowl; mix banana mixture into flour mixture until just combined. Fill muffin cups with batter.

Bake in the preheated oven until a tooth pick inserted in the center of a muffin comes out clean, 30 to 35 minutes.

Whole Wheat Vegan Cinnamon Pancakes

Ingredients
1/2 cup whole wheat flour
1/2 cup rye flour
1 tablespoon soy flour
1 tablespoon white sugar
1 1/2 teaspoons baking powder
1/8 teaspoon salt
1/8 teaspoon ground cinnamon
1/2 teaspoon vanilla extract
1/2 cup water
1/2 cup soy milk
1/4 cup chopped pecans

Directions
In a medium bowl, stir together the whole
wheat flour, rye flour, soy flour, sugar,
baking powder, salt and cinnamon.

Make a well in the center, and pour in the
vanilla, water and soy milk. Mix until all of
the dry Ingredients have been absorbed,
then stir in the pecans.

Heat a large skillet or griddle iron over
medium heat, and coat with cooking
spray. Pour about 1/3 cup of batter onto
the hot surface, and spread out to 1/4 inch
thickness.

Cook until bubbles appear on the surface,
then flip and brown on the other side.
Serve warm.

Zesty Breakfast Couscous

Ingredients
3/4 cup vanilla soymilk
1/4 cup orange juice
1/2 cup dry couscous
1/2 banana, mashed or sliced
1 tsp cinnamon

Directions
In a small pot on high heat bring the "milk" and juice to a boil. Reduce heat and stir in couscous, banana and cinnamon. Cover with lid and simmer for 2-3 minutes.

Turn off heat and let sit for an additional 2 minutes. Serve immediately.

Part 2

Introduction

Nowadays obesity is on the rise. With obesity comes a host of diseases, some more serious than the others, like diabetes, cardiovascular diseases, cancers of different organs, etc. There are many factors that can be attributed to this increase of unhealthy body fat in our bodies, like unhealthy eating habits and lack of exercise.

One of the major contributors of fat in our body is fat that our body gets from the consumption of foods derived from animals. Consumption of red meat, as we all know, is extremely harmful to our health.

A vegan diet, in layman's language, is a diet which avoids the consumption of all meats, eggs and other dairy products.

This book provides you with a brief history of how veganism originated, the reasons why you need to adopt veganism, the benefits, vegan replacements for the commonly used dairy products and eggs, a do's and don'ts guide and of course a bunch of delicious and healthy vegan recipes that will help you kick start your diet.

I would like to thank you for downloading this eBook and hope that the content of this eBook helps pushing you towards a healthier way of life.

Veganism and Its Origin

Veganism basically is a concept that promotes abstinence from any kind of products derived from animals, especially when the diet is concerned. According to Veganism, animals are sentient being and need not be treated as a commodity by us.

Donald Watson, the co-founder of the Vegan Society in England, coined the term "Vegan" in the year 1944 to imply "non-dairy consuming vegetarian". Later on, the word vegan evolved to mean "the principle that a human being should live his or her life without taking undue advantage of helpless creatures.

The concept of vegetarianism has been around since Ancient Greece and India, but the word *vegetarian* came up somewhere around the 19th Century as to refer to those who abstained from meat. The people who did not consume dairy products or eggs were said to be "strict vegetarians" or "total vegetarians."

Vegetarianism picked up in the 19th Century and there were efforts to set up strict vegetarian communities. Around this time the Temple School in Boston, based on strict vegetarian principles.

A lot of publications took up the cause of abstinence from using animal products, highlighting the cruelty against animals. Articles were published asking people to find alternatives for leather shoes and to convert to vegetarianism.

In 1943, Leslie Cross, from the Leicester Vegetarian Society, wrote an article in a newsletter about how she was concerned about the consumption of cow's milk by vegetarianism. You can say that this article set the ball rolling and opened up the gates of Veganism.

In 1944 when their demands for a section in the Vegetarian Society's magazine went unheard, Donald Watson and few other members set up their own quarterly newsletter named the "Vegan News", Watson said in its very first issue that the word vegan was both, the beginning and the end of vegetarianism.

In 1962 the Oxford Illustrated Dictionary defined the word vegan to be *"a vegetarian who eats no butter, eggs, cheese or milk."*

The first vegan society in America came into being in 1948 under the leadership of Catherine T. Nimmo and Rubin Abramowitz.

The American Vegan Society (AVS) was founded in 1960 by H. Jay Dinshah after he visited a slaughterhouse and was inspired by the writings of Donald Watson. He included the Nimmo's society into his and also joined the concept of veganism with the concept of ahimsaa, a Sanskrit word which means "non harming" or "non violence."Even their magazine was named Ahimsa.

In the 1970s veganism was promoted to be a healthier form of diet and a lot of scientists researched and argued that the people who consumed a diet that contained animal fat and proteins were at a greater threat of getting diseases as opposed to people who consumed a low fat plant based diet.

It is difficult to point the exact moment when veganism gained momentum in the 21st Century, but it is believed that the concept gained popularity after T. Colin Campbell's book *The China Study* was released in 2005.

The book talks about the relationship between chronic illnesses, such as cancer, diabetes and coronary heart disease, and consumption of dairy products. Around 2010 and 2011 veganism gained enough momentum in America for restaurants to start marking items as "vegan" on their menus.

The Two Types of Veganism

Yes, veganism is a pretty straightforward concept; live your life without harming any other sentient being. But even this concept can be broadly classified into two types:

Dietary Vegans

Also known as strict vegans, these people refrain from consuming products derived from animals. This is not just limited to avoiding meat, but also extends to dairy products, eggs and all the other products derived from animals, unlike the ovo lacto vegetarians.

Ethical Vegans

These are the people that not only follow a vegan diet, but also avoid all sorts of animal products in other spheres of their lives too, be it for any purpose. This concept is also known as environmental veganism, which is based on the theory that extensive harvesting of animals weakens the ecosystem rendering it unstable.

Reasons For Adopting Vegan Lifestyle

As explained before, veganism has a very great impact on your health. Here are some reasons why you should adopt a vegan lifestyle

Veganism is Healthy

After carrying out various studies during the late 1970s and early 1980s, physicians Caldwell Esselstyn, Dean Ornish, John A. McDougall, Michael Greger, Michael Klaper, Neal D. Barnard and the biochemist T. Colin Campbell argued that an animal fat and protein rich diet can lead to a variety of diseases.

According to T. Colin Campbell in his book "The China Study", consumption of animal fats and proteins gives way to a lot of chronic diseases like the cancer of the bowel, breast and prostate, diabetes and coronary heart disease. He concludes that if people avoid all animal derived foods, like beef, poultry, lamb, beef, eggs and dairy, and consume a diet of plant based foods they can reduce the chances of contracting life threatening diseases.

Veganism is Ethically Correct

After health, "moral grounds" is the second most popular reason why people take up the vegan diet and lifestyle.

Did you know about 25 billion animals are slaughtered in America every year! And the conditions they endure before getting slaughtered are so terrible, you might even think that slaughtering the animal was doing it a favor and relieving it of its misery.

Yes, animals are not intelligent beings (well, according to us humans anyway), but they are sentient. They feel fear and pain as they are rounded up, hoarded in small pens or cages and mercilessly slaughtered, often being left to bleed to death. These half dead animals are often beaten and skinned while there is still life in them!

If you have a pet just take a good look at it and imagine: what if your pet were put through this level of torture?

Many pro-meat eaters say that this is the way of life, part of the food chain cycle and there's nothing wrong with it. Yes, it is not wrong to eat meat. But, it is wrong to eat the meat which comes from an animal, which was provided with disgusting living conditions and was killed without any mercy.

A lot of people, who turn vegan, do so after passing or visiting a slaughterhouse or two. Most people say that one look at that place or even one sniff of that place is enough to make you abstain from meat for life. Give it a thought.

Veganism is Cheaper (Both Immediately and In The Long Run)

A lot of the critics of veganism argue that following a vegan diet is expensive. But let me tell you, this is far from the truth. The fact is that following a vegan diet is a lot cheaper.

First, let us look at how following a vegan diet saves our money on a day to day basis. As we all know the cost of meat is way higher than the cost of a bag of vegetables. The cost of a pound of a regular beef steak costs about $ 2.5 and the cost for prime cuts is even higher. A decent steak of veal costs about $ 14.97 for half a pound.

As compared to this, a pound of tomatoes costs $ 1.47, 10 large russet potatoes cost $ 4 and a pound of red leaf lettuce costs an average $ 3 per pound. While that one piece of steak will make up for one meal, the aforementioned grocery is enough to be used for at least 3 - 4 meals!

The average weekly expenses for a family of four who consume organic and vegan foods is about $ 200, while the average weekly expenses for a family of four who consume meat is about $ 650 - $ 700!

Now, let's talk about the long term monetary benefits of turning vegan. Like mentioned before, consuming vegan foods is extremely healthy. Once you stop consuming the harmful animal fats and proteins, you start protecting your body against a variety of diseases. The consumption of fresh fruits and vegetables results in a consumption of fibers, which help flush the toxins out of your body.

Eating organic and fresh foods also help in boosting your immune system and keep your metabolism running at the optimum level. This saves you a lot of money by reducing your medical expenses.

Veganism Encourages You To "Go Green"

Today, "go green" is a cry that is echoing from every corner of the world. "Go green" is a concept which promotes an environmental friendly and sustainable living.

One of the largest pollutants of America's waterways is animal farming. The wastes generated from animals are often dumped in water bodies or permeate into the ground water table and pollute the drinking water.

When farm animals belch, they release ammonia, which is a major greenhouse gas and plays a major role in global warming! The hooves of farm animals compress the ground and reduce the water holding capacity of the soil and result in more and more water running off the soil.

Also, about 1/3 of the fossil fuels used in America are used on animal harvesting. And when you compare the amount of resources, food, water, infrastructure, etc., devoted to these animal farms and the end product that we receive, the resources far outweigh the end product!

These are just some of the ill effects of excessive animal harvesting and farming.
Do your bit to save the world and stop being the consumer that creates the demand for these animal farms. Remember, once the demand goes down, the numbers of animal farms will go down on their own.

Benefits Of Adopting a Vegan Diet and Lifestyle

Veganism has a lot of advantages and can have a very positive effect on your mind as well as your body.

Nutrition

These are the nutritional benefits that you can derive when you consume a vegan diet consisting of whole grains, fresh fruits, vegetables, soy products, beans and nuts.

1. **Lower Levels of Saturated Fats** – Foods derived from animals like meat cuts

and dairy products are rich in saturated fats and when you consume these foods, you consume a lot of saturated fats. When you stop consuming these foods, you lower your saturated fat content in your body; hence, safeguarding yourself against a variety of cardiovascular diseases.

2. **Fiber** – When you consume fresh fruits and vegetables on a daily basis you consume a high amount of fiber. This fiber is extremely helpful for easy bowel movement and also helps fight the cancer of the colon.

3. **Magnesium** – This nutrient is essential in the absorption of calcium, but is often overlooked. Green leafy vegetables, such as spinach, nuts and seeds have a high amount of magnesium in them.

4. **Calcium** – No, dairy products are not the only source of calcium. Vegan staples like fortified almond milk, soy

milk, broccoli, almonds, kale, turnip, hazel nuts, etc. have a good calcium content and are easier on the digestive system too.

5. **Phytochemicals** – A plant rich diet has a high amount of phytochemicals. These phytochemicals play a major role in preventing and healing cancer, boost the number of protective enzymes and aid the antioxidants in the body.

6. **Proteins** – It is a common misconception that proteins are only present in non vegetarian foods and vegetarians (and by extension vegans) always lack protein in their diet. What is even more uncommonly known is that most Americans eat too much protein and expect proteins from unhealthy sources, like red meat. Soy based products, beans, peas, nuts and lentils, as long as you're not allergic to any of these, are rich healthy sources of protein that have no side effects on

your body (like the consumption of red meat does).

Disease Prevention

We eat food to strengthen our body and provide our body with nutrition that promotes healthy growth. Our food also contains a lot of nutrients that help in protection from the various diseases. Here is a list of some of the diseases that can be prevented, stalled or reversed with the help of a vegan diet and lifestyle.

1. **Cardiovascular diseases** – Like mentioned earlier, when you consume lower levels of saturated fats, you protect your body from cardiovascular diseases. A study done in Britain shows that the risk of getting heart disease reduces with the consumption of vegan food.

2. **Bad Cholesterol** – All food products derived from animals contain varying levels of cholesterol. When you eliminate these foods from your diet

you protect your heart from the effects of cholesterol.

3. **Type 2 Diabetes** – A vegan diet is very effective weapon against type 2 diabetes. Not only does the diet aid in reduction of the risk of getting type 2 diabetes, the diet is a boon for all those who suffer from type 2 diabetes and helps in controlling the disease.

4. **Prostate Cancer** – A study has shown that men, who were in the early stages of prostate cancer, stopped the progress of the disease and, in some cases, even reversed the illness by just switching to a vegan diet and lifestyle.

5. **Colon Cancer** – Studies have shown that people who consume a lot of grains and fresh fruits and vegetables have a lesser chance of contracting colon cancer as opposed to the people who don't.

Physical Benefits

Along with great nutritional benefits and diseases prevention functions, a vegan diet and lifestyle also has many physical advantages. Here are some of the physical benefits of going vegan:

1. **Body Mass Index (BMI)** – BMI is used as an indicator that the individual has the ideal, healthy weight and lacks body fat. Many studies have shown that individuals who stay off meats have a better BMI as compared to those who consume meat.

2. **Weight Loss** – Yes, a lot of diets help in weight loss, but the question is: are they healthy? A vegan diet is one of the healthiest ways to lose weight as the vegan diet eliminates all the unhealthy food and provides you with a diet full of fresh and healthy foods.

3. **Energy** – The main function of food is to provide us with energy. A lot of times, consuming "heavy" fat rich foods has a reverse effect on our body; making us feel more lethargic. A vegan

diet eliminates all those fat rich foods and provides your body with the much needed energy.

4. **Healthy Skin** – The vitamins A and E which we get from the consumption of the vegetables and nuts have a great impact on your skin. It is observed that the people who consume a vegan diet have a healthier and glowing skin as compared to the people who do not follow the vegan diet.

5. **Body Odor** – You may not know this, but if you consume a lot of red meats, there is a high probability of you having body odor issues. When you go vegan you smell better.

6. **Pre Menstrual Syndrome** – Women have reported that they go through a lot less intense and, in some cases, next to negligible PMS symptoms. It is believed that the non consumption of dairy has this effect on the body.

7. **Nails** — Nail health is said to be a reflection of overall health. Consumption of a vegan diet strengthens nails and makes them less prone to chipping.

The Myth Busters — Too Much of the American Diet

A regular American Diet has a lot of food in it. This results in an excessive accumulation of harmful toxins in the body. The list given below outlines how a vegan diet can reduce the problem of excessive food as well as the excessive toxins we consume.

1. **Animal Proteins** — Like mentioned before, a lot of people believe that only animal sources can provide your body with the much needed proteins. This is not true. Beans and grains are a much healthier source of protein, as compared to red meat.

2. **Dairy From Cow's Milk** – Despite what the advertisements running on the television tell us, the fact is that it is very difficult for the human body to digest cow's milk and the various products made using it. According to some studies about 75% of the people in this world may suffer undetected milk allergies or lactose intolerance. When you cut the cow's milk dairy products from your diet, it elevates your overall health.

3. **Mercury** – You will be shocked by the statistics that show the amount of mercury present in the seafood we consume. Varying levels of mercury have been found in fish and shellfish, and it is impossible to consume fish without adding mercury in your body.

Vegan Food Replacements

The vegan diet is pretty much limited to fruits, vegetables, grains, nuts and beans and crosses out almost 50% of the foods available for us. People who are born and brought up vegans may find it very easy to follow the vegan diet, but new converts may find it difficult to adapt to the diet and find replacements for commonly found foods.

A lot of us are so used to consuming dairy products and eggs, when we are faced with the question of what to use as a replacement, we draw up blank. We have provided you with a list of the replacements for the aforementioned foods for a smooth living.

Replacements For Dairy Products

Milk is such a staple part of our lives that most of us non-vegans and non-lactose intolerants can't imagine life without it. After all, without milk, how can you make ice cream? Or as a matter of fact most other desserts?

The answer is very simple; you use supplements. Plant milk, extracted from different plant sources, can be easily used in place for actual milk. Here are a few examples:

- Soy Milk — Soy milk is the most common replacement for regular milk. There is a slight taste difference, but it is next to negligible and can be used for all purposes you usually use milk for.
- Almond Milk — Almond milk can be used as a replacement to almost any recipes where you need milk. So you want a delicious and healthy vegan cake? Just substitute the regular milk for almond milk and not only will it work well, the distinctive almond taste will also add another level of flavor to it.
- Coconut Milk — Like the almond milk, coconut milk also makes a good substitute for milk in the dishes you

need to cook. Coconut cream can also be used as a substitute for dairy cream

If you require cheese you can easily substitute dairy cheese for soy cheese, tapioca cheese or cheese made from nuts.

Margarine can be used to replace regular dairy butter.

Replacements For Eggs

Egg is a very important source of protein and has many functions to perform. Some foods use egg as a binding agent, some as a thickening agent and some as an emulsifying agent.

With so many uses you might think that finding a replacement for eggs might be very difficult, but this is not the case. It is replaceable and you will see how.

Egg free versions of foods (that usually use eggs) are easily available in the market.

For example, eggless mayonnaise is readily available in the market. If you do not wish to buy prepackaged mayonnaise, you can make it at home. Just replace the eggs in the mayonnaise with a handful of flax seeds.

When egg is needed to perform a binding function, say to coat patties before you fry them, replace the egg with some soy flour mixed with water.

Silken tofu can also be used to replace egg in certain recipes.

For baking, substitute eggs with some mashed bananas, apple sauce or mashed prunes.

As you can see, it is possible to replace the non vegan Ingredients with vegan ingredients; all you need to do is some research. Just make sure you get the quantities right so that you are not left with a mess of foul tasting food.

Do's And Don'ts – A Guide To Follow The Vegan Way Of Life

So, after reading the advantages of the vegan diet and lifestyle you have decided you want to go vegan. There are some common mistakes every newly converter vegan does and it is essential that you avoid these at all costs.

Here is a list of do's and don'ts that you should follow to make most of this lifestyle!

The Do's

1. **Get a boost of vitamin B12** – Vitamin B 12 is a really important vitamin which helps maintain our nerve cells and blood cells extremely healthy. The deficiency of this vitamin causes several neurological problems, like demyelination (which leads to tingling sensations and numbness), dementia,

amnesia, mood problems and an uneven gait. This vitamin is mainly found in animal products and this is why most vegans suffer from the deficiency of vitamin B 12.

To safeguard yourself from these diseases make sure you consume at least 25 micrograms of a good quality vitamin B 12 supplement every day.
It is essential that you take your doctor's advice before starting any supplements on your own.

2. **Start off slowly** – Do not get up and decide one day "I'm going to go vegan today." Suddenly switching diets can be a very sudden transition for your body, one which your body may not be able to recover from.
Instead of suddenly starting the vegan diet, make it a slow transition.
Start off as a part time vegan with two vegan meals and one

non vegetarian meal and slowly wean off it over a span of a month.

The Don'ts

1. **Rely on packaged vegan foods** – A lot of the prepackaged vegan meals contain high amounts of sodium and other artificial Ingredients which can be quite detrimental to your health. If you don't believe us, check the calories on a packet of veggie burger patties and the calories on the package of beef burger patties. You will find that the veggie burger patties have a higher calorie content.

    The veggie burger patties may also contain artificial chemicals to provide a good taste, smell and color.
    Do not consume more than a packet of these pre-packaged Vegan foods more than once a week.

2. **Forget about the protein** – It is common knowledge that animal based

foods have a higher protein content as compared to its vegan counterparts. Make sure you consume a protein rich diet to make up for the lost proteins.

Include a lot of soy based products, like soy nuggets, soy milk, tofu, etc., nut based products, like peanut butter, almond butter, etc., quinoa and oatmeal in your daily diet.

3. **Just eat raw food** – A lot of people associate veganism to be synonymous with the consumption of raw foods only. Do not make this mistake of consuming just raw vegetables and fruits. Cooked beans, grains, vegetables and fruits are easier for our body to digest and extract nutrients from. But, this in no way means you need to limit yourself to eating just cooked foods. Create a healthy balance of both cooked and raw foods in your diet. This will not only mix up your diet a bit, but also provide your palate with a variety of textures. Doing so will also break the

monotony of eating similar foods and make you feel excited for meals.

Recipes

Delicious Soba Noodles with Spicy Tahini Sauce, Sea Vegetables and Kale

Ingredients
- 1/4 cup and 2 tablespoons rice vinegar
- 1/4 cup soy sauce
- 2 (8 ounce) packages dried soba noodles
- 1/4 cup olive oil
- 2 bunches kale, torn into bite-sized pieces
- 4 cloves garlic, minced
- 1 teaspoon chili-garlic sauce (such as Sriracha)
- 2 (1.76 ounce) packets Arame seaweed
- 1-1/2 cups tahini
- 1/4 cup water or more as needed
- 2 tablespoons olive oil
- 1/4 cup minced fresh ginger, or to taste

- 1 teaspoon ground turmeric

Method

1. Firstly, add the rice vinegar, tahini, 2 tablespoons olive oil, ground turmeric, soy sauce, 2 tablespoons water and chili-garlic sauce in a large bowl and blend it using a whisk or a fork.
2. Now add water and mix well until the dressing gets a hummus-like consistency.
3. In a pot of lukewarm water soak the arame seaweed for about 15 minutes.
4. Boil the pot of water on medium heat, then drain the seaweed.
5. In a pot boil salted water, cook soba noodles in the same pot until tender.
6. Drain the noodles and set aside.
7. In a large skillet, add the olive oil and heat it over medium-high heat. Now add garlic and cook it until fragrant.
8. Add ginger and drain seaweed to garlic and stir well. Now in the skillet add kale, toss and stir well so the kale is evenly coated.

9. Cover and cook on low heat for 5 to 10 minutes.
10. Now add soba noodles in tahini sauce and toss well until coated.
11. Add the drained seaweed and kale mixture to the noodles and serve.

Avocado Tacos

Ingredients

- 6 avocados - peeled, pitted, and mashed
- 2 bunches fresh cilantro leaves, finely chopped
- 1/2 cup onions, diced
- 24 (6 inch) corn tortillas
- Jalapeno pepper sauce, to taste
- 1/2 teaspoon garlic salt

Method

1. Firstly, heat the oven to 325 degrees F.
2. Now mix the avocados, onions, and garlic salt in a medium bowl.
3. On a baking sheet arrange corn tortillas in a single layer and place it in the

preheated oven for 5 to 10 minutes or until heated through.
4. Add the avocado mixture on the tacos.
5. Sprinkle jalapeno pepper sauce and garnish with cilantro

Banana, Strawberry and Flax Seed Smoothie

Ingredients
- 1 frozen banana, peeled and cut into chunks
- 2 cups frozen strawberries
- 1/4 cup flax seed meal
- 2 cups low-fat vanilla soy milk

Method

1. Place all the Ingredients into a blender. Keep blending until smooth.
2. Pour into tall glasses and serve chilled.

Strawberry, Oatmeal and Soy Milk Breakfast Smoothie

Ingredients

- 2 cups soy milk
- 1 cup rolled oats
- 2 bananas, broken into chunks
- 28 frozen strawberries
- 1 teaspoon vanilla extract
- 1 tablespoon white sugar

Method

1. Firstly, add soy milk, oats, bananas and strawberries in a blender. You can also add vanilla and sugar if desired. Blend it until smooth.
2. Serve chilled in glasses.

Delicious Banana and Kale Smoothie

Ingredients

- 2 bananas
- 4 cups chopped kale
- 1 cup light unsweetened soy milk
- 2 tablespoons flax seeds
- 2 teaspoons maple syrup

Method

1. Place all the Ingredients in a blender.
   Cover the blender and blitz until the
   mixture gets a smoothie like texture.
2. Chill for a few hours or pour it into tall
   glasses over some crushed ice.

Vegan Style Virgin Pina Colada Smoothie

Ingredients
- 6 cubes ice cubes, or as needed
- 2 bananas
- 2 cups fresh pineapple chunks
- 1 cup coconut milk
- 1 cup soy milk
- 2 tablespoons agave nectar
- 2 tablespoons ground flax seed
- 2 teaspoons pure vanilla extract

Method

1. Place all the Ingredients in a blender.
   Now cover it and blend until smooth.
2. Serve the smoothie in a tall glass,
   chilled or pour over some crushed ice
   for immediate serving.

Corn, Peas and Bean Salad

Ingredients
- 1 cup vegetable oil
- 2 cups chopped celery
- 2 (15 ounce) cans of green beans (drained)
- 1 cup chopped green bell pepper
- 2 (15 ounce) cans shoe peg corn (drained)
- 1 cup chopped onion
- 2 (2 ounce) jars pimientos
- 2 cups white sugar
- 2 (15 ounce) cans peas, drained
- 1 teaspoon ground black pepper
- 2 teaspoons salt
- 1-1/2 cups white wine vinegar

Method

1. In a bowl add the peas, corn, green beans, pimentos, celery, bell pepper and onion, mix well.

2. In a sauce pan add the sugar, black
    pepper, salt, oil and vinegar. Now heat
    it and stir well to combine.
3. Bring the mixture to boil and pour it
    over salad.
4. Now mix it well to coat the salad.
5. Refrigerate at least 24 hours.
6. Serve chilled.

Tomato and Olive Salad

Ingredients
- 80 cherry tomatoes, halved
- 2 cups pitted and sliced green olives
- 2 (6 ounce) cans black olives, drained and sliced
- 4 green onions, minced
- 6 ounces pine nuts
- 1 cup olive oil
- 1/4 cup red wine vinegar
- 2 tablespoons white sugar
- 2 teaspoons dried oregano
- Salt, to taste
- Pepper, to taste

Method

1. Combine the cherry tomatoes, green olives, black olives, and green onions in a large bowl.
2. Toast the pine nuts in a dry skillet on medium heat until golden brown. Now stir it into the tomato mixture.
3. Mix oil, red wine vinegar, sugar, and oregano in a small bowl. Add salt and pepper to taste.
4. Now mix it into the salad and stir well to coat evenly.
5. Chill for 1 hour and serve.

Tropical Mango Salad with Walnuts and

Lettuce

Ingredients
- 12 red lettuce leaves, rinsed, dried, and torn
- 6 small mangoes, peeled and cubed
- 1 cup dried cranberries
- 1 cup walnut pieces

- 1 green bell pepper, seeded and thinly sliced
- 1 red bell pepper, seeded and thinly sliced
- 2 carrot, peeled and sliced

Method

1. Add the cranberries, lettuce, red pepper, mangoes, green pepper, carrot and walnuts in a large bowl and toss well.
2. Serve immediately.
3. You can also chill the lettuce beforehand for a delicious tasting salad.

Vegan Style Italian Sweet Potato

Minestrone

Ingredients
- 2 tablespoons vegetable oil
- 10 cloves garlic, minced
- 4 large stalks celery, chopped
- 2 large onion, chopped

- salt and pepper to taste
- 2 (28 ounce) cans Italian-style diced tomatoes
- 4 large carrots, sliced thinly
- 1 tablespoon and 2 teaspoons Italian seasoning
- 10 cups vegetable broth
- 4 large sweet potatoes, peeled and diced
- 3/4 pound green beans, cut into 1 inch pieces

Method

1. In a soup pot, heat the vegetable oil over medium-high heat. Add the celery, salt, onion, pepper and Italian seasoning and sauté for 5 minutes or until tender.
2. Add the vegetable broth, carrots, sweet potatoes, garlic, green bean and tomato (with the juice from the can) and stir well.
3. Boil the mixture and reduce the heat to low, cook until the vegetables are tender or for 30 minutes.

4. Serve immediately.

Delicious Spinach, Potatoes and Baked Mushrooms

Ingredients
- 12 cloves unpeeled garlic
- 1/4 cup olive oil
- 1/2 pound spinach, thinly sliced
- 1 pound Portobello mushrooms
- 2 pounds new potatoes, halved
- 1/4 cup toasted pine nuts
- 2 tablespoons olive oil
- Kosher salt to taste
- Ground black pepper to taste
- 1/4 cup chopped fresh thyme
- 1/2 pound cherry tomatoes

Method
1. Firstly, preheat your oven to 425 degrees F before you start cooking.
2. Add the new potatoes to a shallow roasting pan. Pour about 2 tablespoons

of olive oil on the potatoes and roast the potatoes for about 20 minutes.

3. In an oven safe pan place the mushrooms with their stem side up and garlic. Pour a tablespoon of olive oil on the mushrooms and garlic. Sprinkle some kosher salt and black pepper on it as per your taste. Place the pan in the preheated oven and bake the mushrooms for about 5 – 7 minutes.

4. Remove from oven and add the cherry tomatoes. Again cook in oven until mushrooms are softened or about 5 minutes.

5. Sprinkle the pine nuts on the baked mushrooms and roasted potatoes for an extra crunchy texture.

6. Serve it with sliced spinach.

Vegan Curried Rice

Ingredients

- 1/4 cup olive oil
- 2 tablespoons minced garlic
- 2 tablespoons chili powder

- Black pepper to taste
- 2 tablespoons ground cumin, or to taste
- 2 cubes vegetable bouillon
- 2 cups water
- 2 tablespoons ground curry powder
- 2 tablespoons soy sauce
- 2 cups uncooked white rice

Method

1. Pour some olive oil in a medium sized sauce pan and heat on low heat. Cook the garlic till the garlic releases its aroma and slowly add in the pepper, cumin, curry powder and chili powder.
2. Once the garlic begin to change color and become fragrant, stir in the bouillon cube with a little water.
3. Increase the heat and pour in the remaining water and the soy sauce.
4. Add the rice to the mixture just before the mixture comes to boil. Once the mixture start boiling reduce the heat to low. Cover and cook until the liquid is absorbed or for 15 to 20 minutes.

5. Remove from heat and set aside for 5
    minutes.
6. Serve immediately.

Conclusion

A lot of people have the motto "live to eat" in their lives and eat everything in sight without worrying about the consequences. This is a really wrong behavior and shouldn't be encouraged.

Yes, it is not wrong to enjoy eating food, but anything in excess is pretty harmful.

The vegan diet is an illustrious example of how delicious food can be and healthy too. In this book I have provided you with a variety of reasons why a vegan diet is quite essential and good for your health. I have also provided you with a number of healthy and delicious recipes for you to try at home once you have decided to start converting to a vegan diet and lifestyle.

If after reading this book you have decided to turn vegan, I would like to congratulate you on your healthy and eco-friendly choice. I would just like to remind you that please follow the do's and don'ts outlined in this eBook and please do not start with any medical supplements without consulting your physician. Remember, do it slowly until your body is used to it.

I would like to thank you once again for downloading this book and hope this book helped you make a healthy and environment friendly choice!

About the Author

Jose Smith is author of several cookbooks on Vegan diet. He has written research papers on the topic and currently lives in California.